I'm Going To Lose Weight

NICOLE ESHUN

Copyright © 2015 Nicole Eshun
All rights reserved.

ISBN-13: 978-1514626610

DEDICATION

I would like to dedicate this book to all the people out there who battle with weight loss and esteem issues. I would also like to dedicate 'I'm Going To Lose Weight' to the people who have always wanted to lose weight but lack the will power to do so. I hope this books fills them with motivation.

Contents

1. 5 SIMPLE STEPS
2. 10 WEIGHT LOSS TIPS
3. 7 FOOD IDEAS
4. YOUR GOALS
5. YOUR PLAN
6. FITNESS GAME

5 SIMPLE STEPS

In this chapter I'm going to be telling you what the 5 simple steps to weight loss is. Follow these steps one by one and you will be on your way to a healthier lifestyle, filled with loads of energy.

STEP 1: GET THE RIGHT MIND SET

The key to long term weight loss, along with diet and regular exercise, is a positive mindset that moves you out of an unhealthy past and into a healthier future. harnessing the right outlook that keeps you continually motivated is vital. Whatever we use to lose weight has to be applied long term. Losing weight and maintaining that loss is a lifelong commitment.
Focus on how you can eat nutritious food that fuels your body.

Reflect: Think about how far you have come. Acknowledge that you are successful, and in return success will breed success.

Write everything down: I believe it's an easy way to stay motivated. When you have a bad day, you can go back and look at a good week and see what you did well. At the back of this book we have the option of writing down your fitness and weigh loss goals.

STEP 2: PLAN YOUR MEALS

The further ahead you plan the more clearer your further will be. The same goes for planning your meals.
I've found that preparing myself for tomorrow's meal makes the whole process much easier. Start as soon as you come home from a food shopping trip. Make sure the necessary pots, pans, and dishes for tomorrow's meal are ready so you don't have to do it tomorrow. Have the tools and dry ingredients needed laid out on the counter, so that you can start cooking as soon as you get off from school or work.
Planning out your meals ahead of time can make the whole process much easier, so I recommend giving it a shot—even if you're just doing it with pen and paper a week ahead of time. In chapter 3 there is a 7 day food plan if you get stuck on food ideas.

STEP 3: THE KEY TO SUCCESSFUL WEIGHT LOSS IS APPLYING 75% HEALTHY EATING HABITS AND 25% EXERCISE TO YOUR ROUTINE

Yes, you can lose weight with diet alone, but exercise is an important component. Without it, only a portion of your weight loss is from fat you're also stripping away muscle and bone density. Since working out stimulates growth of those metabolic tissues, losing weight through exercise means you're burning mostly fat. The number on the scale may not sound as impressive, but because muscle takes up less space than fat does, you look smaller and your clothes fit better. Research has shown that to lose weight with exercise and keep it off, you don't need to run marathons. You just need to build up to five to seven workouts a week, 50 minutes each, at a moderate intensity, like brisk walking or Zumba. Resistance training helps, too. But don't just do isolated weight-lifting exercises like biceps curls; you'll get leaner faster by using your body weight against gravity, as with movements like squats, lunges, push-ups and planks. And, of course, beyond burning fat, people shouldn't forget that exercise can have other impressive health perks, like improving the quality of your sleep, lowering your cholesterol and reducing your stress levels.

Many gyms offer a free 1-day pass, you can redeem your free gym pass by going on your local fitness centre's website and filling out a quick form which is just your email and a contact number. Try all your local gyms for free, even bring a date or mate. When you are satisfied with one, join a gym, some start from as little as £10.99 per month.

STEP 4: MORE GREEN MORE LEAN

Your plate should be filled with more vegetables than carbs (rice/bread/pasta)
Take a good, long look at that fast-food cheeseburger.

Every item on it, from the bun to the sauce, was processed in a factory and created in a laboratory. It's packed with enough artificial colours and preservatives to make it look seductive, and enticing.

This is not clean eating. Clean eating is about more than just getting lean; it's about making choices that promote optimum long-term health for your body.

Getting clean might just mean tweaking what you're doing now, or it might require you to turn over a whole new leaf.

No matter if you're a carb-cutter, carb-loader, or intermittent faster, your golden rule of clean eating should be to include as much fresh produce in your daily diet as possible.

Vegetables make every dietary system better and healthier. They provide the vitamins and nutrients to keep you feeling as good as you look, and the soluble fiber to make sure you suck every last bit of nutrition out of everything else you eat.

STEP 5: EVERYTHING IN MODERATION

There are so many healthy options on the market. Such as protein ice creams, protein cookies, brown (wholegrain) rice and brown pasta. When dishing out your food try to eat a fist full of rice/pasta.

The popular belief is that in order to lose weight you must completely eliminate certain foods from your eating habits. Some decide to get rid of sweets, some decide to eliminate starches and others will stop eating meat. By eating in moderation, though, you can learn to lose weight without eliminating any types of food.

Portion Size

One of the biggest problems with eating is that we often eat portion sizes too big, so frequently that we get trained to eat more than we need. Try decreasing your portion size by one-third and you'll find that there isn't much difference. The food will still fill you up as much as usual but the amount of calories taken in will be much lower.

Considerations

Another method of eating in moderation is to completely change your eating schedule. Most people will eat three big meals for breakfast, lunch and dinner. Between each meal the blood sugar drops and it can make you overeat at the next meal. If you learn to eat five or six small meals per day then there isn't enough time between each meal for your blood sugar to drop. These small meals should be meals that are about the size of your fist. I know a few people that set their alarms every three hours for them to eat small meals, or drink a protein shake/meal replacement.

Second Helping

After eating a delicious meal it is common to want to go back and have a second helping. The hungry feeling that you get doesn't always go away immediately. After you have eaten your first helping wait 10 or 15 minutes before going back for a second helping and you may find out that you're not hungry for a second helping after all.

Hydration

Thirst is not always a feeling you get when your mouth is dry and you need something to wet your mouth. Sometimes when you are not hydrated enough you get a feeling in your stomach that is similar to being hungry. If you have that feeling in your stomach and you've already eaten recently then try drinking some water and see if the feeling you are getting is actually thirst.

Warning

Often when people are feeling some kind of emotion they resort to eating. Try not to eat just because you are stressed, sad or because you are bored. Only eat when you are hungry.

Fiber

Foods that are high in fiber, like fruits, are very helpful

to losing weight. Fibre fills you up quicker so that you don't feel hungry but are also low in calories so you are not adding a lot of weight.

Faltering

Sometimes when you try eating in moderation you'll falter and you'll eat a meal that is too big, go back for seconds when you shouldn't or give in to some kind of craving. For some reason when people do this their attitude is to give up and eat poorly the rest of the day or week because they already messed up. **Don't give up**. If you falter sometime during the day then just force yourself to eat something really healthy the next meal and get back on track.

10 WEIGHT LOSS TIPS

Here are 10 quick tips to help you lose weight even faster:

TIP 1: Try dancing every day while getting ready for (work/school) dancing for just 30 minutes a day can burn up to 200 calories.

TIP 2: For extra motivation hire a personal trainer. Try can be booked for as little as £20 per hour/session.

TIP 3: Use Smaller Plates. Learn to control your hunger so that it doesn't control you. create healthy eating habits. Resist processed food. Such foods are toxic sludge.

TIP 4: Drink More Water. Drink plenty of water carry a water bottle where ever you go.

TIP 5: Drink Coffee or Tea.

TIP 6: Eat a High-Protein Breakfast. Eat slowly. Try reading the back of every food packaging as often as possible. Don't just trust want is on the front of the food labels practically the popular brands that say 'Diet' on them. Read the back too. What are the ingredients? A lot of the time they will not be made from natural ingredients.

TIP 7: Keep calm. Don't stress yourself out trying to lose weight. Your body will not cooperate with you if you/it is stressed out. Relaxation and stress release methods such as meditation or prayer if you are religious. Both work well to de-stress you, and keep you balanced.

TIP 8: Take the stairs instead of the lift and try standing up whilst travelling via public transport. By standing rather than sitting for 15 minutes you can burn up to 50 calories. Also while standing up hold your stomach in as much as possible; this will tighten and train your ab muscles.

TIP 9: Replace surgery sweets/snacks with healthier options. Nuts, raisins and grapes are great choices.

TIP 10: Sleep Better.

7 FOOD IDEAS

In this segment you will be given 7 (one week) healthy affordable meal options. This is only a guideline for you to follow. Have a routine. Some people have a strict exercise routine i.e gym five times a weeks, and eating every three hours. The key to successful weight loss is to try and find a routine that works best for you.

MONDAY

Breakfast: Banana porridge Made with water and topped with natural yoghurt, banana, raisins and sweetened with honey.

Lunch: Vegetable soup and oatcakes
Large bowl of vegetable or lentil soup (either homemade or supermarket 'fresh') with oatcakes.

Dinner: Baked salmon with jacket potato
Bake a salmon fillet and serve with a jacket potato and steamed vegetables. Try this meal with **Truffle oil**. Truffle oil is an oil that "seemingly" comes from truffles.

I'm going to eat…

Breakfast _____
_____

Lunch: _____
_____

Dinner: _____
_____

TUESDAY

Breakfast: Fresh fruit and yoghurt
Fresh fruit and a pot of natural yoghurt sweetened with honey.

Lunch: Piri piri lamb
With wholegrain rice salad

Dinner: Chicken curry

I'm going to eat…

Breakfast _____
_____

Lunch: _____
_____

Dinner: _____
_____

WEDNESDAY

Breakfast: Muesli and yoghurt
Homemade muesli made from oats, seeds, nuts and dried fruit served with natural yoghurt.

Lunch: Fish and chips
With homemade potatoes chips

Dinner: Quorn cottage pie

I'm going to eat…

Breakfast _____

Lunch: _____

Dinner: _____

THURSDAY

Breakfast: One wholegrain toast and beans

Lunch: Grilled salmon
With salad

Dinner: Soba noodles With tofu and mushrooms

I'm going to eat…

Breakfast _____
_____

Lunch: _____
_____

Dinner: _____
_____

FRIDAY

Breakfast: Tomato and basil omelets

Lunch: Jacket potato with grilled cod
Grilled cod fillet served with jacket potatoes and lightly steamed vegetables.

Dinner: Tuna and prawns with noodles
Gently fry a selection of vegetables such as onions, mushrooms, peppers, courgette and leek in a little olive oil.

I'm going to eat…

Breakfast _____
_____

Lunch: _____
_____
Dinner: _____
_____

SATURDAY

Breakfast: Granola cereal Packed full of nuts, fruit and seeds

Lunch: Avocado and prawn salad
Fresh avocado served with prawns, salad, balsamic vinegar and lemon juice.

Dinner: Tuna and sweet corn jacket potato
Jacket potato topped with tuna (canned in water) mixed with sweetcorn

I'm going to eat...

Breakfast _____
_____

Lunch:_____
_____

Dinner: _____
_____

SUNDAY

Breakfast: Vegetarian fry-up Made with fresh organic eggs and have a crusty baguette on hand to soak up the delicious sauce.

Lunch: Easy Mushroom Quiche

Dinner: Chinese vegetable stir fry
Stir fry a selection of vegetables such as bok choi, spring onions, mushrooms, bamboo shoots and beansprouts in a little olive oil with garlic and ginger. Serve with brown rice.

I'm going to eat...

Breakfast _____
_____

Lunch: _____
_____

Dinner: _____
_____

Healthy snacks

Natural yoghurt mixed with honey

Handful of unsalted nuts or seeds

Fresh fruit or fresh fruit salad

Plain popcorn

Rice cakes

Green tea

Granola

I'M GOING TO LOSE WEIGHT

YOUR GOALS

The more you give yourself reasonable goals and achieve them successfully, the more you will keep that habit.
Write your fitness goals down

1. _____
2. _____
3. _____
4. _____
5. _____
6. _____
7. _____
8. _____
9. _____
10. _____

YOUR PLAN

How do you plan on achieving your fitness goals?
What steps will you take?

1. _____
2. _____
3. _____
4. _____
5. _____
6. _____
7. _____
8. _____
9. _____
10. _____

FITNESS GAME

What do you need to get right in order to have a long term weight loss?

_____

Success will breed?

_____

Why is meal planning important?

_____

What is the formula to successful weight loss results

75% _____
25% _____

Write down healthy options for snacks

_____
_____
_____
_____
_____
_____

For further health and fitness tips download the game: Jump Over Garbage (JOG) from Google Play.

www.ingramcontent.com/pod-product-compliance
Lightning Source LLC
Chambersburg PA
CBHW072315200526
45168CB00014B/1652